The Best Slow Cooker Recipes for Women Over 40

The best cookbook for Beginner and Advanced Users on a Budget

Shirley M. Griffin

Sommario

Beans & Grains Recipes 5

INTRODUCTION

Hello there! Welcome to my publication of recipes for the Crockery Pot.

My recipes are merely too tasty to maintain to myself. As well as it's the only recipe book you'll require to make the most tasty Crock Pot recipes you've ever tasted!

If there's one kitchen device I can't live without, it's my Crockery Pot. This gizmo has actually changed my life entirely in the cooking area! Gone are the days when I spent hours each week, prepping and after that cooking dishes. And so sometimes those meals were tasteless, with leftovers that nobody intended to eat.

Then along came my Crockery Pot Pressure Cooker ... as well as currently I make delightful meals on a daily basis.

One of the most significant enticing features of the Crock Pot is that it makes fresh and also fast cozy dishes quickly. Whether you're vegetarian or like your meat and also hen, my publication has the very best recipes for making incredible, healthier meals. As well as see to it you make an elegant rip off recipe on those days when you're not counting calories and also fat! Those are the best recipes of all. In this book, I share my favored.

Chives Cabbage Petals

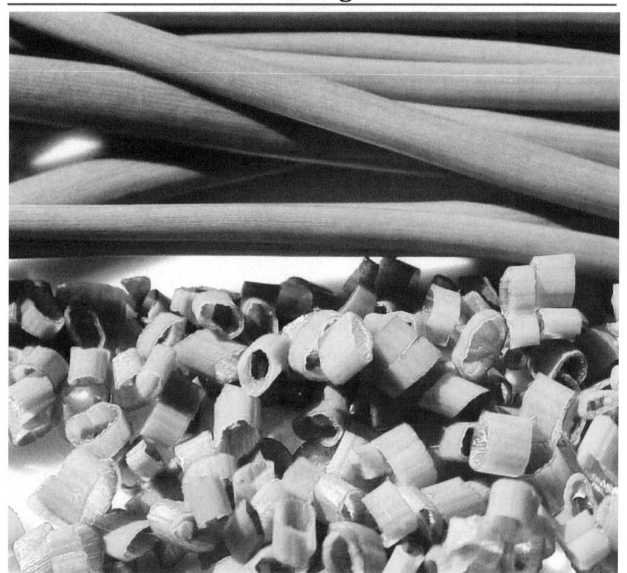

Prep time: **10 minutes**

Cooking time: **15 minutes**

Servings: **4**

Ingredients

- 1-pound cabbage
- 1 tablespoon chives
- 1 bell pepper, chopped
- 1 teaspoon salt
- 1 teaspoon white pepper
- ¾ cup of water
- ½ cup almond milk

Directions:

1. **Cut the cabbage into the petals. Cut every petal into 4 pieces and place in the pressure cooker.**
2. **Sprinkle the vegetables with chives, chopped bell pepper, salt, white pepper, and almond milk.**
3. **Add water and stir gently. Close the lid.**
4. **Cook the cabbage on the steam mode for 15 minutes.**
5. **When the time is over, open the lid and stir the petals gently. Transfer them in the serving bowls.**

Nutrition: **calories 108, fat 7.4, fiber 4.1, carbs 10.9, protein 2.5**

Garlic Beans with Pecans

Prep time: **10 minutes**

Cooking time: **10 minutes**

Servings: **8**

Ingredients

- 14 ounces green beans
- 5 ounces pecans
- 1 cup of water
- 1 tablespoon minced garlic
- 4 ounces raisins
- 1 teaspoon salt
- 1 tablespoon butter
- ¼ teaspoon curry

Directions:

1. **Cut the green beans into halves, sprinkle them with the garlic, raisins, salt, and curry and mix well.**
2. **Crush the pecans and combine them with the green beans mixture. Pour the water in the pressure cooker.**
3. **Transfer the green beans mixture in the trivet and place the trivet in the pressure cooker.**
4. **Close the lid and cook at "Steam" mode for 10 minutes.**

5. When the time ends, transfer the dish to a serving plate. Add the butter and mix Well before serving.

Nutrition: **calories 190, fat 14.5, fiber 3, carbs 16.21, protein 3**

Lemon Onion Rings

Prep time: **5 minutes**

Servings: **4**

Ingredients

- 3 big white onions
- 1 tablespoon liquid stevia
- 1 tablespoon lemon juice
- 1 teaspoon lemon zest
- 1 tablespoon butter
- 1 teaspoon ground white pepper
- ¼ cup of soy sauce
- 1 teaspoon ground ginger

Directions:

1. **Combine the liquid stevia, lemon juice, lemon zest, butter, ground white pepper, ground ginger, and soy sauce and mix well.**

2. **Peel the onions and slice them.**

3. **Make rings from the onions and transfer them to the sweet mixture. Place the sliced onions in the pressure cooker.**

4. Add the soy sauce mixture. Close the pressure cooker lid and cook for 5 minutes on "Pressure" mode.

5. When the cooking time ends, remove the cooked onion rings from the pressure cooker. Let the dish rest briefly and serve.

Nutrition: **calories 83, fat 3.1, fiber 2.8, carbs 12.6, protein 2.4**

Carrot Half and Half Soufflé

Prep time: **10 minutes**

Cooking time: **25 minutes**

Servings: **7**

Ingredients

- 5 big carrots, boiled
- 1 cup coconut flour
- ⅓ cup half and half
- ½ cup cream
- 1 teaspoon vanilla sugar
- ½ teaspoon cinnamon
- ⅓ cup erythritol
- ½ teaspoon baking soda
- 1 tablespoon apple cider vinegar
- 1 tablespoon butter
- 1 teaspoon ground anise

Directions:

1. **Mash the carrots using a blender. Combine the carrots with the coconut flour, half and half, cream, vanilla**

sugar, cinnamon, Erythritol, baking soda, apple cider vinegar, butter, and ground anise.

2. Mix until smooth.
3. Place the carrot mixture in the pressure cooker.
4. Close the lid and cook at "Steam" mode for 25 minutes. When the cooking time ends, let the soufflé rest briefly and serve.

Nutrition: **calories 133, fat 6..2, fiber 7.1, carbs 16, protein 3.2**

Red Pepper Green Beans

Prep time: **10 minutes**

Cooking time: **4 minutes**

Servings: **5**

Ingredients

- 15 oz green beans, chopped
- 1 tablespoon olive oil
- 1 teaspoon salt
- 1 teaspoon red pepper
- 1 cup water, for cooking

Directions:

1. **Pour water in the cooker and add green beans.**
2. **Close the lid and cook them onhigh-pressure mode for 5 minutes. Then make quick pressure release and open the lid.**
3. **Drain water and transfer the green beans in the ice water to save their color. After this, return the green beans back in the cooker.**
4. **Sprinkle them with olive oil, salt, and red pepper.**

5. **Stir gently and close the lid. Set air crisp mode and cook the meal for 4 minutes (380F) or until the vegetables are light crispy.**

Nutrition: **calories 58, fat 3, fiber 3.2, carbs 7.9, protein 1.8**

Cauliflower Rice Bell Peppers

Prep time: **5 minutes**

Cooking time: **10 minutes**

Servings: **9**

Ingredients

- 1 cup cauliflower rice, cooked
- 10 ounces green bell pepper
- ½ cup cottage cheese
- 1 tablespoon paprika
- ½ teaspoon salt
- 1 teaspoon onion powder
- 1 cup chicken stock
- ½ cup sour cream
- 1 teaspoon olive oil
- 1 large onion
- 1 tablespoon cilantro

Directions:

1. Remove the seeds from the bell peppers.

2. Combine the cauliflower rice, cottage cheese, paprika, salt, onion powder, sour cream, and cilantro and stir well.

3. Peel the onion and dice it. Set the pressure cooker to "Sauté" mode. Pour the olive oil in the pressure cooker and add the onion.

4. Sauté the diced onion for 2 minutes. Add the cooked onion to the cottage cheese mixture and stir it.

5. Fill the bell peppers with the cottage cheese mixture and place them on the trivet. Transfer the trivet in the pressure cooker and close the lid.

6. Cook and cook on "Steam" mode for 10 minutes.

7. When the cooking time ends, remove the dish from the pressure cooker and let it rest briefly. Serve the stuffed peppers warm.

Nutrition: **calories 99, fat 4, fiber 2.7, carbs 13.9, protein 4.1**

Artichoke Stew

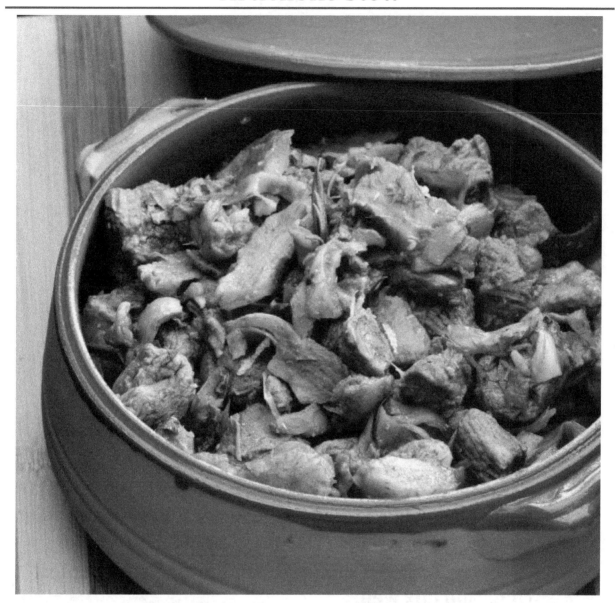

Prep time: **10 minutes**

Cooking time: **11 minutes**

Servings: **5**

Ingredients

- 1 pound artichoke
- 1 teaspoon red chile flakes
- 1 teaspoon of sea salt
- 1 teaspoon oregano
- 1 white onion
- 1 cup pork rinds
- ¼ cup wine
- 6 ounces Parmesan cheese
- 2 garlic cloves
- 1 teaspoon fresh dill

Directions:

1. **Chop the artichoke and sprinkle it with the red chile flakes and sea salt. Add oregano and dill and mix well.**
2. **Pour the wine in the pressure cooker. Add garlic cloves and artichokes. Close the pressure cooker lid and cook for 10 minutes at the "Pressure" mode.**
3. **Grate the Parmesan cheese, combine it with the pork rinds and mix well.**
4. **When the artichokes are cooked, strain them and combine them with the cheese mixture.**
5. **Mix well and cook it on "Pressure" mode for 1 minute.**
6. **Release the pressure and open the pressure cooker lid. Transfer the cooked dish to a serving bowl.**

Nutrition: **calories 366 fat 19.5, fiber 5.6, carbs 13.8, protein 35.9**

Asparagus Tart

Prep time: **10 minutes**

Servings: **8**

Ingredients

- 7 ounces keto soda dough
- 10 ounces asparagus
- ⅓ cup walnuts
- 3 tablespoons butter
- 1 teaspoon salt
- 1 teaspoon ground black pepper
- ⅓ cup tomato paste
- 1 onion
- 1 carrot
- 1 egg yolk

Directions:

1. **Roll out the dough using a rolling pin.**
2. **Spread the pressure cooker with the butter inside and place the rolled dough. Chop the asparagus and transfer it to the blender.**

3. Add the walnuts, salt, ground black pepper, tomato paste, and egg yolk. Peel the onion and carrot. Grate the carrot and chop the onion.

4. Add the onion in a blender and puree until smooth. Combine the asparagus mixture with the carrot and mix well.

5. Spread the dough with the asparagus mixture.

6. Close the pressure cooker lid Cook at "Pressure" mode for 25 minutes.

7. When the cooking time ends, release the pressure and open the pressure cooker lid. Transfer the tart to a serving plate, cut into pieces, and serve.

Nutrition: **calories 191, fat 9.2, fiber 5.4, carbs 11.8, protein 17.5**

Spinach Tarts

Prep time: **10 minutes**

Servings: **8**

Ingredients

- 6 ounces butter
- 1 cup coconut flour
- 1 teaspoon salt
- ½ teaspoon Erythritol
- 3 cups spinach
- ½ cup sour cream
- 1 teaspoon ground white pepper
- ½ tablespoon oregano
- 1 teaspoon cayenne pepper

Directions:

1. **Chop the butter and combine it with the coconut flour and salt. Add Erythritol and knead the dough.**
2. **Roll the dough out and place it in the pressure cooker. Chop the spinach and combine it with the sour cream.**

3. Sprinkle the mixture with ground black pepper, oregano, and cayenne pepper. Mix well and spread it on the dough.

4. Close the pressure cooker lid Cook at "Pressure" mode for 15 minutes. When the cooking time ends, let the tart rest briefly.

5. Transfer the tart to a serving plate, slice it and serve.

Nutrition: **calories 248, fat 22.4, fiber 5.5, carbs 9.5, protein 3**

Lettuce Wraps

Prep time: **10 minutes**

Servings: **5**

Ingredients

- 7 ounces lettuce
- 1 white onion
- 1 eggplant
- 5 ounces mushrooms
- 1 tablespoon olive oil
- ½ tablespoon salt
- 1 teaspoon butter
- ½ teaspoon red chile flakes
- ½ teaspoon cayenne pepper
- 1 tablespoon fresh basil

Directions:

1. **Peel the onion and chop it. Chop the eggplant into tiny pieces. Combine the chopped vegetables together in a mixing bowl.**

2. Chop the mushrooms and add them to the mixture. Sprinkle the mixture with the salt, red chile flakes, and cayenne pepper and mix well.

3. Add the basil and mix again. Add the butter to the pressure cooker and add olive oil. Preheat the mixture at the "Sauté" mode for 3 minutes.

4. Add the eggplant mixture and cook for 15 minutes on "Pressure" mode.

5. When the vegetable mixture is cooked, remove it from the pressure cooker and let it rest.

6. Place the vegetable mixture in the middle of the lettuce leaves and wrap it. Serve immediately.

Nutrition: **calories 157, fat 4.1, fiber 8, carbs 31.02, protein 5**

Beef Asparagus Mash

Prep time: **10 minutes**

Cooking time: **10 minutes**

Servings: **5**

Ingredients

- 3 cups beef broth
- 16 ounces asparagus
- 1 tablespoon butter
- 1 teaspoon cayenne pepper
- ½ teaspoon chile pepper
- 1 tablespoon sriracha
- 2 teaspoons salt
- ⅓ cup sour cream
- 1 teaspoon paprika

Directions:

1. **Wash the asparagus and chop it roughly. Place the chopped asparagus in the pressure cooker.**
2. **Add cayenne pepper and beef broth.**
3. **Add salt and close the pressure cooker lid.**

4. Cook the dish for 10 minutes at the "Pressure" mode. Remove the asparagus from the pressure cooker and strain it.

5. Place the asparagus in a food processor.

6. Add chile pepper, butter, sriracha, and sour cream. Blend the mixture until smooth.

7. Place the cooked asparagus mash in the serving bowl.

Nutrition: **calories 72, fat 4.5, fiber 2, carbs 5.14, protein 4**

Mushrooms Vegetable Stew

Prep time: **10 minutes**

Cooking time: **25 minutes**

Servings: **10**

Ingredients

- 2 eggplants
- 2 yellow sweet pepper
- 1 zucchini
- 1 cup green beans
- 8 ounces mushrooms
- 1 tablespoon salt
- ½ teaspoon ground black pepper
- 1 cup chicken stock
- 3 cups beef broth
- ½ cup tomato juice
- 1 tablespoon Erythritol

Directions:

1. **Peel the eggplants and chop them. Sprinkle the chopped eggplants with the salt and stir the mixture.**
2. **Remove the seeds from the sweet peppers.**

3. Chop the sweet peppers and zucchini. Combine all the ingredients together in the mixing bowl.

4. Add Erythritol and mix up the mixture.

5. Place the vegetable mixture in the pressure cooker and sauté it for 5 minutes, stirring frequently.

6. Add tomato juice, beef broth, chicken stock, green beans, and mix well. Close the pressure cooker lid Cook at "Sauté" mode for 25 minutes.

7. When the stew is cooked, let it rest briefly and serve.

Nutrition: **calories 61, fat 0.9, fiber 5.1, carbs 11.4, protein 4.1**

Creamy Chile Peppers

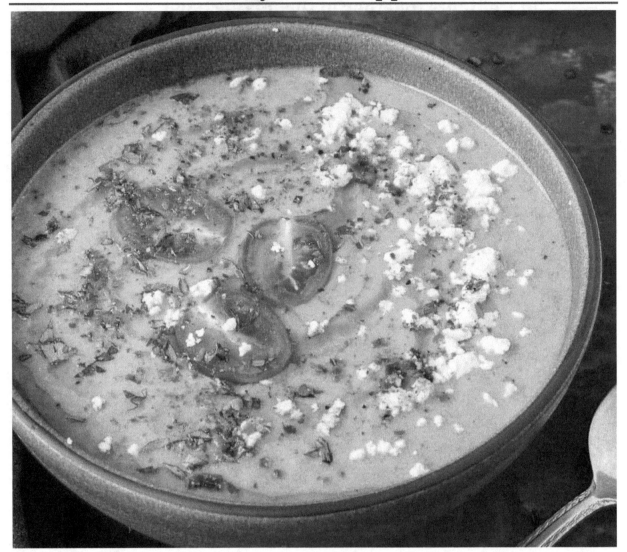

Prep time: **10 minutes**

Cooking time: **10 minutes**

Servings: **5**

Ingredients

- 5 chile peppers
- ½ cup half and half

- ⅓ cup olive oil
- 1 cup coconut flakes
- 1 teaspoon cilantro
- ¼ cup coconut flour
- 1 egg
- 1 teaspoon ground thyme

Directions:

1. **Remove the seeds from the chile peppers and combine them with the coconut flour. Beat the egg in the bowl.**
2. **Sprinkle the chile peppers with the whisked egg. Add the coconut flakes, cilantro, and ground thyme and mix well.**
3. **Pour the olive oil in the pressure cooker and preheat it well. Add the chile peppers to the pressure cooker and roast them at "Sauté" mode for 8 minutes on both sides.**
4. **When the chile peppers are cooked, remove them from the pressure cooker, let it rest briefly, and serve.**

Nutrition: **calories 221, fat 22.6, fiber 1.9, carbs 4.4, protein 2.5**

Red Cabbage with Raisins

Prep time: **10 minutes**

Servings: **4**

Ingredients

- 10 oz red cabbage, shredded
- ½ cup of water
- 1 oz raisins, chopped
- 1 teaspoon paprika
- 1 teaspoon ground coriander
- 1 teaspoon ground cinnamon
- ½ teaspoon apple cider vinegar
- ½ cup heavy cream

Directions:

1. **Place red cabbage in the cooker.**
2. **Sprinkle it with the paprika, ground coriander, ground cinnamon, apple cider vinegar, and raisins. Add heavy cream and mix up the mixture. Then add water.**
3. **Close the lid and cook the meal on saute mode for 30 minutes.**

4. Stir it from time to time. The cooked cabbage will have a soft texture.

Nutrition: **calories 94, fat 5.7, fiber 2.5, carbs 10.9, protein 1.5**

Oregano Turnip

Prep time: **10 minutes**

Cooking time: **6 minutes**

Servings: **6**

Ingredients

- 1 pound turnip, boiled
- 1 cup fresh oregano
- 1 egg
- ¼ cup coconut flour
- 1 teaspoon onion powder
- 1 tablespoon salt
- 4 tablespoons olive oil
- 1 teaspoon nutmeg
- 1 teaspoon dill

Directions:

1. **Mash the turnip carefully using a fork or masher. Mince the oregano and add it to the potatoes. Beat the egg into the mixture.**

2. **Sprinkle it with the coconut flour, onion powder, nutmeg, and dill. Knead the dough.**

3. Pour the olive oil in the pressure cooker and preheat it on "Steam" mode.

4. Make medium-sized croquettes from the turnip mixture and put them in the pressure cooker.

5. Cook the croquettes for 6 minutes on each side until golden brown.

6. Remove the croquettes from the pressure cooker, drain them on the paper towel to remove any excess oil and serve.

Nutrition: **calories 155, fat 11.6, fiber 6.8, carbs 13.6, protein 3.1**

Parmesan Zucchini Balls

Prep time: **10 minutes**

Servings: **6**

Ingredients

- 7 ounces Parmesan
- 2 zucchini
- 1 teaspoon salt
- 1 egg
- 1 teaspoon ground black pepper
- ½ cup coconut flour
- 3 tablespoons butter
- ¼ cup parsley

Directions:

1. **Grate the zucchini, sprinkle it with the salt and ground black pepper, and mix well. Grate the Parmesan cheese.**
2. **Beat the egg in the separate bowl and whisk it.**
3. **Add the whisked egg in the zucchini mixture and add the cheese. Chop the parsley and add it to the zucchini mixture.**
4. **Add the coconut flour and knead the dough that forms.**

5. Make small balls from the zucchini mixture and place them on the trivet. Transfer the trivet with the zucchini balls into the pressure cooker.

6. Cook at "Steam" mode for 15 minutes.

7. When the zucchini balls are cooked, remove them from the pressure cooker and serve.

Nutrition: **calories 185, fat 13.9, fiber 1.3, carbs 4.5, protein 12.7**

Tomato Jam

Prep time: **10 minutes**

Servings: **5**

Ingredients

- 10 ounces tomatoes
- 1 tablespoon fresh basil
- ½ teaspoon cinnamon
- ½ cup Erythritol
- ½ teaspoon ground ginger
- 1 tablespoons nutmeg
- 1 tablespoons butter
- 1 teaspoon anise

Directions:

1. **Wash the tomatoes carefully and chop them.**
2. **Combine the basil, cinnamon, Erythritol, ground ginger, nutmeg, and anise and mix well.**
3. **Put the chopped tomatoes in the pressure cooker and add the spice mixture.**

4. Add the butter and mix well. Cook the dish on the "Sauté" mode for 20 minutes. When the cooking time ends, open the pressure cooker lid and stir the jam.

5. Transfer the jam to a serving dish and let it cool before serving.

Nutrition: **calories 39, fat 2.9, fiber 1.1, carbs 3.2, protein 0.7**

Jalapeno Peppers Crisps

Prep time: **10 minutes**

Servings: **5**

Ingredients

- 5 jalapeno peppers, sliced
- 1/3 cup coconut flour
- 2 eggs, whisked
- 1 teaspoon salt
- 1 teaspoon olive oil

Directions:

1. **In the mixing bowl, combine together whisked eggs and salt.**
2. **Then add sliced jalapeno peppers and mix up. After this, coat jalapeno slices in the coconut flour generously.**
3. **Transfer the jalapeno slices in the cooker and sprinkle with olive oil. Close the lid and cook them on air crisp mode for 5 minutes (380F).**
4. **Stir them well and cook for 2-3 extra minutes if jalapeno slices are not crispy enough.**

Nutrition: **calories 71, fat 3.7, fiber 3.8, carbs 6.5, protein 3.5**

Cremini Mushrooms with Paprika

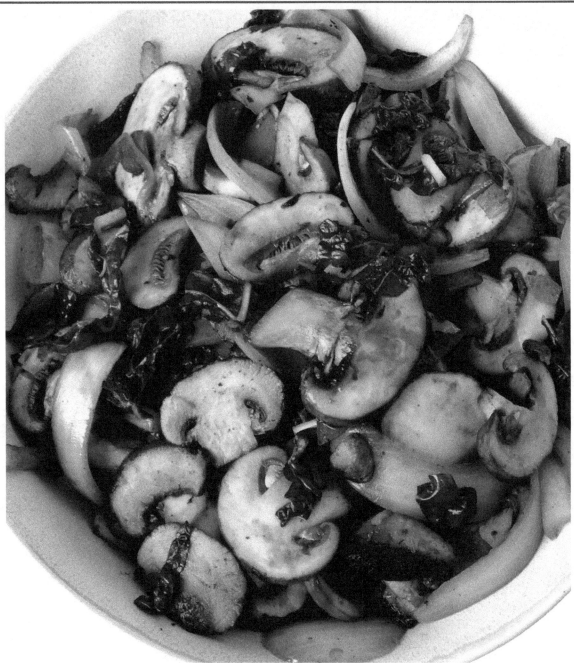

Prep time: **10 minutes**

Cooking time: **7 minutes**

Servings: **5**

Ingredients

- 1 tablespoon turmeric
- 1 pound cremini mushrooms
- 1 cup sour cream
- 1 onion
- 1 tablespoon paprika
- 3 tablespoons olive oil
- 1 teaspoon salt
- ½ teaspoon cayenne pepper

Directions:

1. **Peel the onions and dice them. Pour the olive oil in the pressure cooker and add the onions.**

2. **Set the pressure cooker to "Sauté" mode. Sauté the onion for 3 minutes, stirring frequently.**

3. **Chop the mushrooms and combine them with the paprika, salt, and cayenne pepper and mix well.**

4. **Add the chopped cremini mixture in the pressure cooker and cook it for 2 minutes more. Add the sour cream and mix well. Add turmeric and stir again.**

5. **Close the pressure cooker Cook at "Pressure" mode for 2 minutes.**

6. **When the cooking time ends, release the pressure and open the pressure cooker. Transfer the cooked dish to a serving bowl.**

Nutrition: **calories 422, fat 14.2, fiber 12, carbs 75.79, protein 11**

Rutabaga and Beans Chili

Prep time: **15 minutes**

Servings: **12**

Ingredients

- 5 ounces rutabaga
- ¼ teaspoon cayenne pepper
- 1 teaspoon salt
- ½ teaspoon ground black pepper
- 8 ounces tomatoes
- 1 cup black beans, cooked
- 1 carrot
- 2 eggplants
- 1 teaspoon olive oil
- 1 teaspoon oregano
- 3 cup chicken stock

Directions:

1. **Peel the rutabagas and dice them. Set the pressure cooker to "Sauté" mode. Pour the olive oil in the pressure cooker.**

2. Add the rutabaga and sauté it for 5 minutes.

3. Meanwhile, chop the tomatoes and eggplants. Combine the cayenne pepper, salt, ground black pepper, and oregano in a mixing bowl.

4. Peel the carrot and grate it. Combine all the vegetables together and sprinkle them with the spice mixture.

5. Mix well and place it in the pressure cooker.

6. Add the chicken stock and black beans. Mix well and close the pressure cooker lid. Cook at "Sauté" mode for 20 minutes.

7. When the cooking time ends, remove the dish from the pressure cooker. Rest briefly and serve.

Nutrition: **calories 94, fat 1, fiber 6.4, carbs 18, protein 4.9**

Shepherd's Pie

Prep time: **15 minutes**

Servings: **7**

Ingredients

- 2 white onions
- 1 carrot
- 10 ounces cauliflower mash
- 3 ounces celery stalk
- 1 tablespoon salt
- 1 teaspoon paprika
- 1 teaspoon curry
- 1 tablespoon tomato paste
- 3 tablespoons olive oil

Directions:

1. **Peel the carrot and grate it. Chop the celery stalk.**
2. **Combine the vegetables together and mix well. Put the vegetable mixture in the pressure cooker. Add the paprika, curry, tomato paste, olive oil, and salt.**
3. **Mix well and stir well. Cook at "Pressure" mode for 6 minutes, stirring frequently.**

4. Spread the vegetable mixture with the cauliflower mash and close the pressure cooker lid. Cook the dish on the "Pressure" mode for 10 minutes.

5. When the cooking time ends, release the pressure and open the pressure cooker lid. Transfer the pie to a serving plate, cut into slices and serve.

Nutrition: **calories 107, fat 9.3, fiber 2.3, carbs 6.2, protein 1.6**

Thyme Burgers

Prep time: **10 minutes**

Servings: **8**

Ingredients

- 1 cup black soybeans, cooked
- 1 onion
- 1 carrot
- 1 cup fresh thyme
- ⅓ cup spinach
- ¼ cup coconut flour
- 1 egg
- 1 tablespoon salt
- 1 teaspoon ground black pepper
- 1 teaspoon Dijon mustard
- 3 tablespoons starch

Directions:

1. Wash the thyme and spinach and chop them.

2. Place the thyme and spinach in the blender and add the lentils. Blend the mixture for 1 minute. Transfer the mixture to a mixing bowl.

3. Sprinkle it with the coconut flour, egg, salt, ground black pepper, Dijon mustard, and starch. Peel the onion and carrot and grate the vegetables.

4. Add all the vegetables to the thyme mixture and mix well. Make medium-sized "burgers" from the mixture.

5. Place the burgers in the trivet and transfer the trivet in the pressure cooker. Cook at "Steam" mode for 15 minutes.

6. When the burgers are cooked, let them rest briefly, and transfer them to a serving plate.

Nutrition: **calories 155, fat 5.8, fiber 5.1, carbs 17.2, protein 10.1**

White Celery Fries

Prep time: **10 minutes**

Cooking time: **8 minutes**

Servings: **2**

Ingredients

- 6 oz celery root, peeled
- 1 teaspoon white pepper
- Cooking spray

Directions:

1. **Cut the celery root into fries and sprinkle them with the white pepper. Mix up well the vegetables and transfer in the Foodi cooker basket.**
2. **Spray the fries with the cooking spray gently and close the lid.**
3. **Cook the fries at 385F on air crisp mode for 8 minutes. Stir the fries after 4 minutes of cooking.**

Nutrition: **calories 38, fat 0.3, fiber 1.8, carbs 8.5, protein 1.4**

Cinnamon Pumpkin Puree

Prep time: **10 minutes**

Servings: **5**

Ingredients

- 1 pound sweet pumpkin
- 2 cups of water
- 1 tablespoon butter
- 1 teaspoon Erythritol
- 1 teaspoon cinnamon
- ½ teaspoon ground black pepper
- ¼ teaspoon nutmeg

Directions:

1. **Peel the pumpkin and chop it. Put the chopped pumpkin in the pressure cooker. Add the water and ground pepper.**
2. **Close the pressure cooker lid Cook at "Pressure" mode for 10 minutes.**
3. **Strain the pumpkin and place it in a food processor.**

4. **Add Erythritol, butter, cinnamon, and nutmeg. Blend the mixture until smooth. Transfer the pumpkin puree to serving bowls.**

Nutrition: **calories 233, fat 8.7, fiber 2, carbs 38.28, protein 3**

Creamy Onions Soup

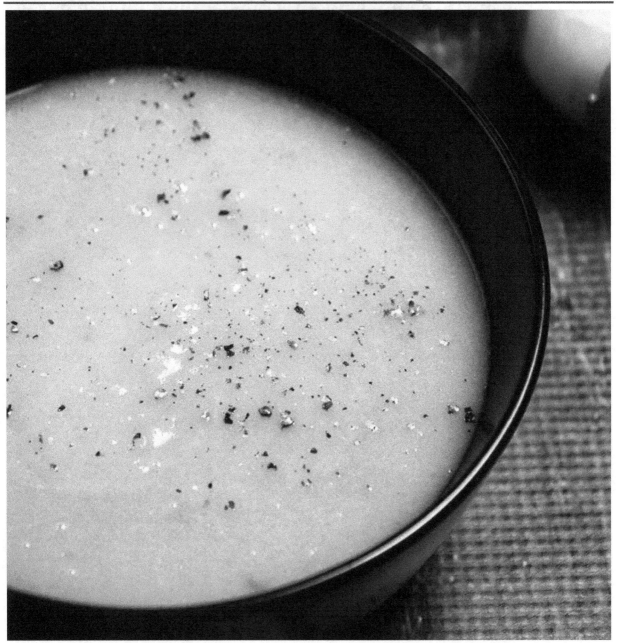

Prep time: **10 minutes**

Cooking time: **15 minutes**

Servings: **14**

Ingredients

- 5 onions
- 1 cup cream
- 3 cups chicken stock
- 1 tablespoon salt
- 1 teaspoon olive oil
- 2 tablespoons butter
- ½ tablespoon ground black pepper

Directions:

1. **Peel the onions and grate them.**
2. **Place the onions in the pressure cooker. Add the olive oil and sauté the onion for 5 minutes, stirring frequently.**
3. **Add the salt, chicken stock, cream, butter, and ground black pepper. Cook at "Pressure" mode for 10 minutes.**
4. **When the soup is cooked, ladle it into serving bowls. Serve.**

Nutrition: **calories 47, fat 3.1, fiber 0.9, carbs 4.5, protein 0.8**

Turmeric Carrot Bites

Prep time: **10 minutes**

Servings: **7**

Ingredients

- 5 carrots
- 1 cup coconut flour
- ⅓ cup whey
- 1 teaspoon baking soda
- 1 tablespoon lemon juice
- 1 teaspoon salt
- 1 teaspoon cilantro
- ½ teaspoon turmeric
- 1 tablespoon olive oil
- 1 teaspoon nutmeg

Directions:

1. **Peel the carrots and grate them.**
2. **Combine the grated carrot with the coconut flour, whey, baking soda, lemon juice, salt, cilantro, turmeric, and nutmeg. Knead the dough.**

3. Make a long log and cut it into small pieces. Set the pressure cooker to "Sauté" mode. Pour the olive oil in the pressure cooker.

4. Make small pieces from the carrot mixture and put them in the pressure cooker.

5. Sauté the carrot bites for 5 minutes or until the carrot bites are golden brown on all sides.

6. Transfer the carrot bites to the paper towel to drain the excess oil and let them rest before serving.

Nutrition: **calories 115, fat 4.5, fiber 6.9, carbs 15.5, protein 3**

Parsnips Risotto

Prep time: **10 minutes**

Servings: **5**

Ingredients

- 4 ounces parsnips
- 1 cup cauliflower rice
- 1 teaspoon salt
- 3 cups chicken stock
- 1 tablespoon turmeric
- ½ cup green peas
- 1 teaspoon paprika
- 2 carrots
- 1 onion
- ½ teaspoon sour cream

Directions:

1. **Chop the parsnip. Peel the onion and carrots.**
2. **Chop the vegetables into the tiny pieces and combine them with the parsnip. Sprinkle the vegetable mixture with the salt, turmeric, paprika, and sour cream.**

3. Place the vegetable mixture in the pressure cooker and cook it at the "Pressure" mode for 6 minutes, stirring frequently.

4. Add the cauliflower rice, green peas, and chicken stock and mix well using a wooden spoon.

5. Close the pressure cooker Cook at "Slow Cook" mode for 20 minutes.

6. When the cooking time ends, open the pressure cooker lid and stir well. Transfer the dish to serving bowls.

Nutrition: **calories 65, fat 0.8, fiber 3.9, carbs 13.3, protein 2.5**

Brussel Sprouts Balls

Prep time: **10 minutes**

Cooking time: **10 minutes**

Servings: **2**

Ingredients

- 1 cup Brussel Sprouts
- 1 teaspoon olive oil
- ½ teaspoon ground black pepper
- 5 oz bacon, sliced

Directions:

1. **Mix up together sliced bacon with olive oil and ground black pepper.**
2. **Then wrap every Brussel sprout in the bacon and transfer in the Foodi cooker basket. Secure the balls with toothpicks, if needed.**
3. **Close the lid and set air crisp mode. Cook the meal for 10 minutes at 375F.**
4. **Stir the balls during cooking from time to time. Transfer the cooked balls in the serving bowls.**

Nutrition: **calories 424, fat 32.1, fiber 1.8, carbs 5.4, protein 27.8**

Chopped Asparagus Saute

Prep time: **15 minutes**

Servings: **4**

Ingredients

- 2 cups asparagus, chopped
- 2 garlic cloves, diced
- ½ cup heavy cream
- ½ cu of water
- 1 teaspoon butter
- 1 teaspoon ground turmeric
- 1 teaspoon salt

Directions:

1. **Place asparagus in the cooker.**
2. **Add diced garlic, butter, ground turmeric, salt, and heavy cream. Mix up the mixture until it gets an orange color.**
3. **Then add water and stir it gently again.**
4. **Close the lid and set Saute mode. Cook the asparagus saute for 35 minutes.**

5. **When the time is over, switch off the cooker and let asparagus rest for 15 minutes.**

Nutrition: **calories 78, fat 6.7, fiber 1.6, carbs 3.9, protein 1.9**

Prep time: **15 minutes**

Cooking time: **25 minutes**

Servings: **9**

Ingredients

- 2 green zucchini
- 2 eggplants
- 1 cup tomatoes
- 3 green bell peppers
- 4 garlic cloves
- 2 red onion
- 1 cup tomato juice
- 1 teaspoon olive oil
- 1 cup chicken stock
- 1 teaspoon ground black pepper

Directions:

1. **Slice the zucchini and eggplants. Slice the tomatoes.**
2. **Remove the seeds from the bell peppers and slice them. Peel the onions and garlic cloves. Chop the onions and garlic.**

3. Combine tomato juice, olive oil, chicken stock, and ground black pepper together in the mixing bowl.

4. Place the sliced vegetables to the pressure cooker. Sprinkle the mixture with the onion and garlic.

5. Pour the tomato juice mixture and close the pressure cooker lid. Cook at "Steam" mode for 25 minutes.

6. When the cooking time ends, remove the dish from the pressure cooker. Let it rest briefly and serve.

Nutrition: **calories 82, fat 1.4, fiber 6, carbs 16.53, protein 4**

Green Pea Stew

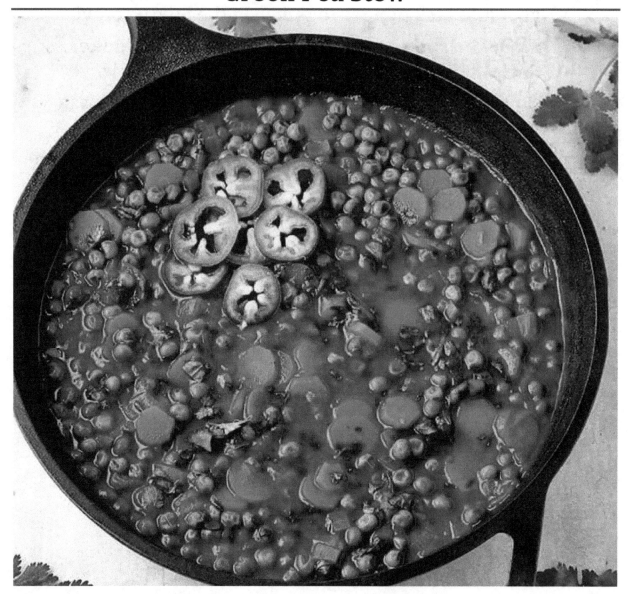

Prep time: **10 minutes**

Cooking time: **35 minutes**

Servings: **6**

Ingredients

- 2 cup green peas

- 1 tablespoon salt
- 4 cups chicken stock
- 1 carrot
- 1 tablespoon olive oil
- 7 ounces ground chicken
- ⅓ cup tomato juice
- ⅓ teaspoon cilantro

Directions:

1. **Peel the carrot and chop it roughly. Put the chopped carrot in the pressure cooker and sprinkle it with the olive oil.**
2. **Cook the carrot at the "Pressure" mode for 5 minutes. Add the green peas.**
3. **Sprinkle the mixture with the salt, chicken stock, ground chicken, tomato juice, and cilantro and mix well.**
4. **Close the pressure cooker lid Cook at "Sauté" mode for 30 minutes.**
5. **When the stew is cooked, let it rest briefly. Transfer the cooked stew to serving bowls.**

Nutrition: **calories 171, fat 7.4, fiber 3, carbs 13.72, protein 13**

Squash Saute

Prep time: **10 minutes**

Servings: **6**

Ingredients

- 2 cups Kabocha squash, chopped
- 1 teaspoon ground cinnamon
- 1 teaspoon curry paste
- 1 teaspoon curry powder
- ½ teaspoon dried cilantro
- 1 cup of water
- 1 tablespoon pumpkin seeds, chopped
- 1 tablespoon butter
- ¾ cup heavy cream

Directions:

1. **Place squash in the cooker and sprinkle it with ground cinnamon, curry powder, and dried cilantro.**
2. **Add butter, water, and pumpkin seeds.**
3. **After this, in the separated bowl, mix up together heavy cream with the curry paste. Pour the liquid in the cooker and mix up well.**

4. Close and seal the lid. Cook the saute for 10 minutes on high-pressure mode.

5. Then allow natural pressure release for 15 minutes. Open the lid and transfer kabocha squash and gravy in the serving bowls.

Nutrition: **calories 97, fat 8.7, fiber 0.8, carbs 4.5, protein 1.2**

Creamy Leek Soup

Prep time: **10 minutes**

Servings: **7**

Ingredients

- 10 ounces leek
- 2 garlic cloves
- 5 cups vegetable stock
- 1 teaspoon salt
- 1 yellow onion
- 1 tablespoon olive oil
- ⅓ cup sour cream
- 1 teaspoon oregano
- 4 ounces noodles
- 1 teaspoon butter
- 1 teaspoon ground white pepper

Directions:

1. **Chop the leek. Peel the garlic cloves and slice them. Peel the onion and dice it. Combine the onion and garlic.**

2. Mix well and place it in the pressure cooker. Set the pressure cooker to "Sauté" mode. Add butter and sauté for 7 minutes.

3. Add chopped leek and pour the vegetable stock. Sprinkle the soup mixture with the salt, ground white pepper, oregano, and cream.

4. Close the pressure cooker lid Cook at "Sauté" mode for 10 minutes.

5. Open the pressure cooker lid and add the noodles. Mix the soup well and close the pressure cooker lid.

6. Cook at "Pressure" mode for 2 minutes.

7. Release the pressure and open the pressure cooker lid. Stir the soup well, then ladle the soup into serving bowls.

Nutrition: **calories 155, fat 5.9, fiber 1, carbs 19.47, protein 6**

Basic Veggie Stew

Prep time: **15 minutes**

Servings: **7**

Ingredients

- 2 carrots
- 1 zucchini
- 8 ounces broccoli
- 4 ounces cauliflower
- 4 cups chicken stock
- ¼ cup tomato paste
- 1 teaspoon sugar
- ½ tablespoon salt
- ⅓ cup parsley
- 1 tablespoon butter
- 2 onions
- 1 teaspoon oregano

Directions:

1. **Wash the broccoli and cut it into florets. Chop the zucchini and carrots.**

2. Place the vegetables in the pressure cooker.

3. Add the chicken stock and tomato paste. Sprinkle the mixture with the sugar, salt, butter, and oregano.

4. Mix well and close the pressure cooker lid. Cook at "Sauté" mode for 10 minutes. Peel the onions and chop them roughly.

5. When the cooking time ends, open the pressure cooker lid and add the onions. Chop the parsley and add it to the stew mixture.

6. Add butter and mix well.

7. Close the pressure cooker lid Cook at "Pressure" mode for 10 minutes.

8. When the stew is cooked, release the pressure and open the lid. Mix the stew carefully. Add the stew to serving bowls.

Nutrition: **calories 71, fat 2.3, fiber 3.2, carbs 11.7, protein 3**

Cheese Baked Asparagus

Prep time: **10 minutes**

Ingredients:

- 9 oz asparagus
- 1 teaspoon garlic powder
- ½ cup heavy cream
- ¼ cup of water
- ½ cup Mozzarella, grated
- 1 teaspoon dried oregano
- ¼ teaspoon salt

Directions:

1. Chop the asparagus roughly.

2. In the mixing bowl combine garlic powder with heavy cream, water, salt, and dried oregano.

3. Then pour the liquid in the instant pot and preheat it on sauté mode for 5 minutes.

4. After this, add chopped asparagus and Mozzarella.

5. Close the lid and cook the meal on manual mode (high pressure) for 1 minute.

6. When the time is over, make the quick pressure release.

Nutrition value/serving: **calories 78, fat 63, fiber 1.6, carbs 3.8, protein 2.9**

Creamy Brussels Sprouts

Prep time: **10 minutes**

Ingredients:
- 6 oz Brussels sprouts
- 1/3 teaspoon salt
- ½ teaspoon ground black pepper
- 1 teaspoon butter
- ½ cup heavy cream

Directions:

1. Melt butter in sauté mode and add Brussels sprouts.

2. Sprinkle them with salt and ground black pepper and cook on sauté mode for 3 minutes.

3. Stir the vegetables and add heavy cream.

4. Close the lid and cook the meal on manual mode (high pressure) for 3 minutes.

5. When the cooking time is finished, allow the natural pressure release for 10 minutes.

6. Stir the vegetables before serving.

Nutrition value/serving: **calories 106, fat 8.9, fiber 2.2, carbs 5.9, protein 2.4**

Turmeric Bacon Carrot

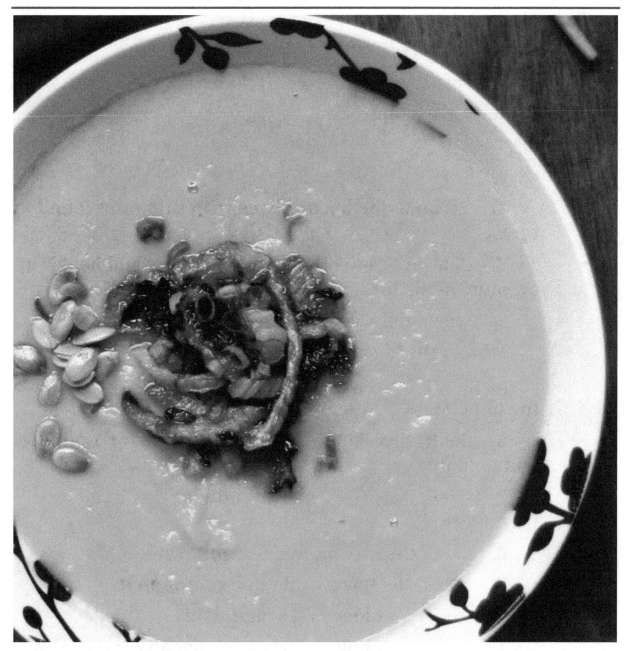

Prep time: **15 minutes**

Cooking time: **4 minutes**

Servings: **3**

Ingredients:
- 2 large carrots, peeled

- 3 bacon slices
- ¾ teaspoon salt
- ¼ teaspoon ground turmeric
- 1 teaspoon avocado oil
- 1 cup water, for cooking

Directions:

1. Sprinkle the bacon slices with salt and ground turmeric.

2. Pour avocado oil in the instant pot and heat it up on sauté mode for 2 minutes.

3. Meanwhile, cut the carrots into 6 pieces.

4. Cut the bacon into 6 pieces too.

5. Wrap every carrot piece in the bacon and put in the hot oil in one layer.

6. Cook the vegetables on sauté mode for 1 minute and then flip on another side.

7. Cook the carrot for 1 minute more. Then transfer in the plate.

8. Clean the instant pot and add water.

9. Insert the trivet and put a carrot on it.

10. Close and seal the lid.

11. Cook the wrapped bacon carrot for 2 minutes.

12. Then make the quick pressure release.

Nutrition value/serving: **calories 102, fat 7.2, fiber 1.3, carbs 4.9, protein 5.4**

Caprese Zoodles

Prep time: **15 minutes**

Servings: **6**

Ingredients:
- 1 zucchini, trimmed
- ½ cup cherry tomatoes, halved
- ½ cup mozzarella cheese, balls
- 1 teaspoon fresh basil, chopped
- 1 tablespoon lemon juice
- ¼ teaspoon white pepper
- 1 teaspoon sesame oil
- 1 cup water, for cooking

Directions:

5. **Pour water in the instant pot and insert the steamer rack.**

6. **With the help of the spiralizer make the noodles from the zucchini and put them in the steamer rack.**

7. **Close and seal the lid and set the timer on "0".**

8. **Cook the zucchini on high pressure.**

9. **When the cooking time is finished, make the quick pressure release and open the lid.**

10. **Transfer the zucchini noodles in the big salad bowl.**

11.   Add cherry tomatoes, mozzarella balls, and basil.

12.   Then sprinkle the ingredients with lemon juice, white pepper, and sesame oil.

13.   Shake the meal gently.

Nutrition value/serving: **calories 22, fat 1.3, fiber 0.6, carbs 1.9, protein 1.2**

Cauliflower and Broccoli Florets Mix

Prep time: **10 minutes**

Cooking time: **4 minutes**

Servings: **3**

Ingredients:

- ½ cup cauliflower florets
- ¼ cup broccoli florets
- 1 tablespoon hazelnuts
- ¼ teaspoon minced garlic
- 1 tablespoon avocado oil
- 1/3 teaspoon salt
- 1 cup water, for cooking

Directions:

10. **Pour water and insert the steamer rack in the instant pot.**

11. **Put the cauliflower florets and broccoli florets in the steamer.**

12. **Close and seal the lid. Cook the vegetables on manual mode (steam mode) for 4 minutes.**

13. **When the cooking time is finished, make the quick pressure release and open the lid.**

14. **Cool the vegetables to the room temperature and transfer in the big bowl.**

15.	Chop the hazelnuts and add in the vegetables.

16.	Then sprinkle the ingredients with minced garlic, avocado oil, and salt.

17.	Shake the well.

Nutrition value/serving: **calories 23, fat 1.6, fiber 1, carbs 2, protein 0.8**

Faulkland Brussels Sprouts

Prep time: **10 minutes**

Cooking time: **7 minutes**

Servings: **3**

Ingredients:

- ¼ teaspoon Erythritol
- 1 teaspoon balsamic vinegar
- 2 tablespoons sesame oil
- ¼ teaspoon salt
- ¼ teaspoon chili flakes
- 8 oz Brussels sprouts
- 1 cup water, for cooking

Directions:

7. Pour water and insert the steamer rack in the instant pot.

8. Put Brussels sprouts in the steamer rack and close the lid.

9. Cook them on steam mode for 2 minutes. Then make the quick pressure release and open the lid.dan the instant pot.

10.   Remove the steamer rack.

11.   Pour the sesame oil in the instant pot and heat it up on sauté mode for 3 minutes.

12.   Add cooked Brussels sprouts.

13.   Then sprinkle the vegetables with balsamic vinegar, chili flakes, and salt.

14.   Stir them and cook for 2 minutes.

Nutrition value/serving: **calories 113, fat 9.3, fiber 2.8, carbs 6.9, protein 2.6**

Soft Sautéed Vegetables

Prep time: **10 minutes**

Cooking time: **8 minutes**

Servings: **4**

Ingredients:
- ½ cup radish, sliced
- 1 green bell pepper, chopped
- 1 zucchini, chopped
- 1 teaspoon tomato paste
- ½ teaspoon salt
- ½ teaspoon ground coriander
- 3 tablespoons avocado oil
- 1 cup water, for cooking

Directions:

8. **In the shallow bowl mix up avocado oil and tomato paste.**

9. **Pour water and insert the trivet in the instant pot.**

10. **In the mixing bowl combine radish, bell pepper, and zucchini.**

11. **Sprinkle the vegetables with salt and ground coriander.**

12. **Then add tomato paste mixture. Stir the vegetables.**

13.   After this, transfer them in the instant pot baking pan and cover with foil.

14.   Put the baking pan on the trivet and close the lid.

15.   Cook the vegetables on manual mode (high pressure) for 8 minutes.

16.   Then make the quick pressure release.

Nutrition value/serving: **calories 35, fat 1.5, fiber 1.7, carbs 5.2, protein 1.2**

Cumin Squash Nests

Prep time: **20 minutes**

Cooking time: **5 minutes**

Servings: **4**

Ingredients:

- 12 oz spaghetti squash, peeled
- 1 egg, beaten
- ¼ teaspoon salt
- 1 tablespoon coconut flour
- ¼ teaspoon ground cumin
- 1 cup water, for cooking

Directions:

8. **Grate the spaghetti squash and mix it up with egg, salt, coconut flour, and ground cumin.**

9. **After this, fill the muffin molds with a grated squash mixture. Flatten the mixture in the shape of a nest. Use the spoon for this step.**

10. **Pour water and insert the steamer rack in the instant pot.**

11. **Arrange the muffin molds with squash nests and close the lid.**

12. **Cook the meal on manual (high pressure) for 5 minutes.**

13. **Then make the quick pressure release.**

14. Remove the cooked squash nests from the muffin molds.

Nutrition value/serving: **calories 50, fat 1.9, fiber 0.6, carbs 7, protein 2.2**

Buttery Green Beans

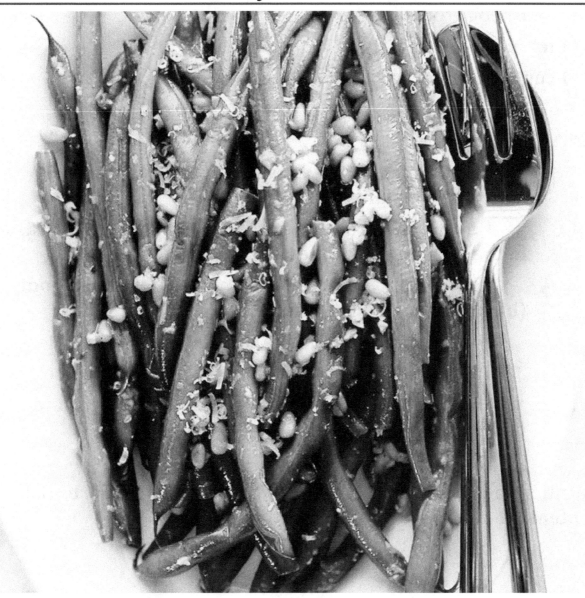

Prep time: **10 minutes**

Cooking time: **1 minute**

Servings: **3**

Ingredients:

- 8 oz green beans, chopped
- 1 teaspoon dried lemongrass

- 1 teaspoon lime juice
- ¼ teaspoon ground nutmeg
- 1 teaspoon butter, melted
- 1 cup water, for cooking

Directions:

11.	Pour water and insert the steamer rack in the instant pot.

12.	Place the green beans and lemongrass in the rack and close the lid.

13.	Cook the vegetables on manual mode (high pressure) for 1 minute.

14.	Then make the quick pressure release.

15.	Transfer the green beans in the bowl.

16.	Add lime juice, ground nutmeg, and melted butter. Stir the vegetables well.

Nutrition value/serving: **calories 37, fat 1.4, fiber 2.6, carbs 5.8, protein 1.4**

Cucumbers and Zucchini Noodles

Prep time: **10 minutes**

Cooking time: **minute**

Servings: 4

Ingredients:

- 2 cucumbers
- 1 zucchini, trimmed
- 1 teaspoon fresh dill, chopped
- 1 garlic clove, diced
- 1 teaspoon fresh parsley, chopped
- 1 tablespoon olive oil
- ¼ teaspoon chili powder
- 1 cup water, for cooking

Directions:

9.   Make the noodles from zucchini and put them in the steamer rack.

10.   Pour water and insert the steamer rack in the instant pot. Close the lid.

11.   Cook the vegetable noodles for 1 minute on steam mode. Then make a quick pressure release and transfer the zucchini noodles in the salad bowl.

12.   Make the spirals from the cucumbers and add them to the zucchini.

13. Then add dill, diced garlic, parsley, olive oil, and chili powder.

14. Gently stir the ingredients.

Nutrition value/serving: **calories 99, fat 0.7, fiber 4.4, carbs 22.8, protein 2.7**

Eggs and Mushrooms Cups

Prep time: **10 minutes**

Cooking time: **7 minutes**

Servings: **4**

Ingredients:

- 1 cup white mushrooms, grinded
- 2 eggs, beaten
- 2 tablespoons almond flour
- ¼ teaspoon salt
- ¼ teaspoon dried thyme
- 1 teaspoon cream cheese
- 1 teaspoon sesame oil
- 1 cup water, for cooking

Directions:

8. **In the mixing bowl mix up grinded mushrooms, eggs, almond flour, salt, thyme, and cream cheese.**

9. **Then brush the muffin molds with sesame oil.**

10. **Put the mushroom mixture in the muffin molds.**

11. **Then pour water and insert the trivet in the instant pot.**

12. **Put the muffin molds on the trivet and close the lid.**

13. **Cook the meal on manual mode (high pressure) for 7 minutes.**

14.   Then make the quick pressure release.

15.   The meal tastes the best when it is cooled to the room temperature.

Nutrition value/serving: **calories 128, fat 10.7, fiber 1.7, carbs 3.8, protein 6.4**

Italian Verde Skillet with Nuts

Prep time: **10 minutes**

Cooking time: **1 minute**

Servings: **4**

Ingredients:

- 2 cups Italian dark leaf kale
- 1 teaspoon peanuts, chopped
- 1 teaspoon hazelnuts, chopped
- 1 teaspoon apple cider vinegar
- 1 tablespoon cream cheese
- ½ teaspoon salt
- 1 cup water, for cooking

Directions:

7. **Pour water in the instant pot.**

8. **Chop the kale roughly and put it in the steamer rack.**

9. **Arrange the steamer rack in the instant pot and close the lid.**

10. **Cook the kale on manual mode (steam mode) for 1 minute. Then make the quick pressure release.**

11. **Transfer the kale in the bowl.**

12. **Add apple cider vinegar, cream cheese, and salt.**

13. Then add hazelnuts and peanuts and mix up the meal well.

Nutrition value/serving: **calories 35, fat 1.8, fiber 1.4, carbs 3.7, protein 2.3**

Shredded Squash with Bacon

Prep time: **20 minutes**

Servings: **8**

Ingredients:

- 4 oz bacon, chopped
- 1-pound spaghetti squash
- 1 tablespoon sesame oil
- 1 teaspoon salt
- 1 cup water, for cooking

Directions:

8. Pour water and place trivet in the instant pot.

9. Wash and clean the spaghetti squash. Then cut it into halves and put in the trivet.

10. Close the lid and cook it on manual mode (steam mode) for 8 minutes.

11. Then allow the natural pressure release for 15 minutes.

12. Then transfer the spaghetti squash in the plate. Shred it with the help of the fork.

13. After this, transfer the shredded squash meat in the salad bowl.

14. Clean the instant pot and remove the trivet.

15.   Add chopped bacon and cook it on sauté mode for 7 minutes. Stir it from time to time.

16.   Add the cooked bacon in the shredded spaghetti squash.

17.   Then add salt and sesame oil. Stir it.

Nutrition value/serving: **calories 109, fat 7.9, fiber 0, carbs 4.1, protein 5.6**

Cilantro and Green Peas Salad

Prep time: **10 minutes**

<u>Cooking time:</u> **3 minutes**

Servings: **2**

Ingredients:

- ½ cup green peas, frozen
- ½ teaspoon fresh cilantro, chopped
- ½ teaspoon avocado oil
- ¼ teaspoon ground paprika
- ¾ teaspoon salt
- ½ cup white cabbage, shredded
- 1 cup water, for cooking

<u>Directions:</u>

10.   **Pour water and insert the steamer rack in the instant pot.**

11.   **Place the green peas in the steamer rack and close the lid.**

12.   **Cook it on the steam mode (high pressure) for 3 minutes. Allow the natural pressure release for 5 minutes.**

13.   **Transfer the cooked green peas in the bowl.**

14.   **Add cilantro, avocado oil, ground paprika, salt, and white cabbage.**

15.   **Stir the salad well.**

Nutrition value/serving: **calories 36, fat 0.4, fiber 2.4, carbs 6.5, protein 2.2**

Organic Risotto

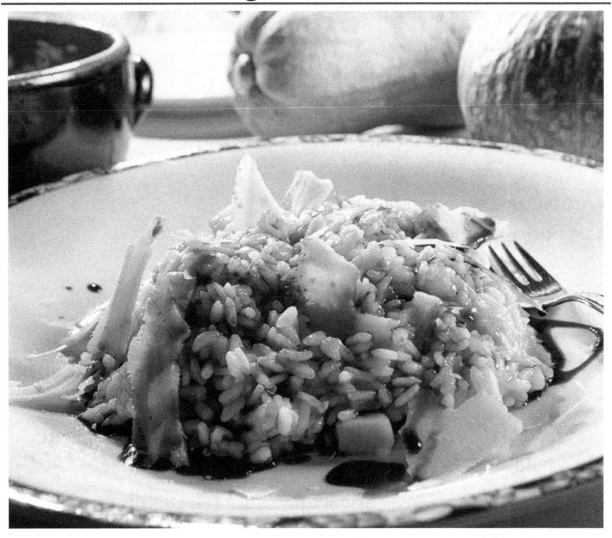

Prep time: **10 minutes**

Cooking time: **16 minutes**

Servings: **4**

Ingredients:

- 2 cups cauliflower, shredded
- 1 teaspoon coconut oil
- ¼ cup white onion, diced
- 6 oz white mushrooms, chopped
- ¼ teaspoon garlic powder
- ½ cup of organic almond milk
- 1/3 cup chicken broth
- 1 teaspoon coconut flour
- ½ teaspoon salt

Directions:

9. **Put the coconut oil in the instant pot. Heat up it on sauté mode for 2 minutes.**

10. **Then add onion, mushrooms, garlic powder, and salt.**

11. **Stir it and sauté for 10 minutes.**

12. **After this, add chicken broth and almond milk.**

13. **Add cauliflower and mix up the risotto.**

14. **Close the lid and cook it on manual mode (high pressure) for 4 minutes.**

15. **Then make the quick pressure release.**

16. **Stir the risotto well.**

Nutrition value/serving: **calories 46, fat 1.9, fiber 2.2, carbs 5.4, protein 3.1**

Collard Greens with Cherry Tomatoes

Prep time: **15 minutes**

Cooking time: **5 minutes**

Servings: **4**

Ingredients:
- 3 cups collard greens, chopped
- ½ cup cherry tomatoes, halved
- ½ red onion, diced
- 1 teaspoon avocado oil
- ½ teaspoon chili flakes
- ¼ oz Parmesan, grated
- 1 cup water, for cooking

Directions:

9. Pour water and insert the steamer rack in the instant pot.

10. Place the chopped collard greens in the rack and close the lid.

11. Cook the greens on manual (high pressure) for 5 minutes.

12. When the cooking time is finished, allow the natural pressure release for 10 minutes.

13. Transfer the cooked collard greens in the salad bowl.

14.	Add cherry tomatoes and diced red onion.

15.	Shake the ingredients gently.

16.	Then add chili flakes and avocado oil, and Parmesan.

17.	With the help of two spoons or spatulas, mix up the meal.

Nutrition value/serving: **calories 26, fat 0.8, fiber 1.7, carbs 4.2, protein 1.7**

CONCLUSION

We have actually come to the end of this great and also plentiful Crockery Pot pressure cooker.

Did you get a kick out of trying these new and tasty recipes?

We truly desire so, in addition to much more will turn up promptly.

To emphasize the remodellings, constantly integrated with our scrumptious as well as also healthy and balanced as well as balanced dishes of exercise, this is a pointers that we intend to use because we consider it the most efficient mix.

A massive hug in addition to we will certainly be back soon to keep you company with our recipes. See you quickly.

CPSIA information can be obtained
at www.ICGtesting.com
Printed in the USA
LVHW061055180521
687737LV00004B/245